THE GREAT LOVER

Make love like a male pornstar

Nazeem Nour

Disclaimer

Although in this book you will only find natural and risk free advices and suggestions, the author of this book is not responsible for any incident that might happen after following the steps. If you suffer from any condition or if you have doubts, please consult a practitioner before following the advices of this book.

Introduction

After several years of research on sexual energy, I decided to write this book to share my knowledge and to help you become better in bed. The topic of sexual energy fascinates me because of its importance and also because of the pleasure it brings .The good lover can change your life especially if you're not good in bed. You will find joy and satisfaction that only even money can not bring you, especially if you suffer from sexual issues like premature ejaculation or impotence...

This e-book will help you improve your level of performance in bed slowly but surely .I do not promise you a magic formula that can have dangerous side effects! But a solid method, natural and based on ancient Taoist knowledge.

This method will not only enable you to become the best in bed, but it will allow you to feel good in your body and in life in general .The sex affects not only your love life but also all other aspects of life .It can improve your career, your social life by giving you more confidence.

This book is intended not only to those who suffer from sexual problem (erectile dysfunction, impotence, premature ejaculation, frequent nocturnal ejaculation ...) .But also to the one who wants to increase his sexual energy and enjoy a fulfilling sexuality throughout his life.

You should know that we each have our own sexual energy. Some of us are born with more energy than others and they are good in bed, others with less sexual energy and might unfortunately suffer from sexual problems, impotence, premature ejaculation ....But the good news is that no matter in which category you find yourself you can improve your sexual life and this book will show you exactly how to be the best lover your partner have ever known.

Even if you're already good in bed, you can still improve it .you will learn how to maintain the sexual energy you have and even increase.

This method is the result of years of reading on the subject of sex. It is based on Taoists sexual teachings. You should know that in Taoist sexual energy is so important, they have developed a method that preserves ejaculation called "sexual Kung Fu" .This method was secretly passed from one person to another until it was revealed to the public many years ago.

With the method contained in this book you'll not only increase your sexual energy and learn how to make love controlling your ejaculation .you'll also improve your overall health, increase your energy and enjoy life, friends and family but you'll also attract many good things .It is possible that your salary increases and this for the simple reason that money and linked to sexual energy. Studies have found a link between money and sexual energy. Napoleon Hill the author of the bestselling book of all time devotes an entire chapter in his famous book "think and grow rich" where he reveals that it is essential to grow the sexual energy to attract abundance. Among all rich men he studied during the 35 years of research, he found that these men had a greater sexual energy.

It's a shame that today we are not taught the importance of sex life, and how sex is closely related to all aspects of our life and that success depends on energy and sexual energy.

This book is divided into two parts .In the first I show you how to increase/maintain your sexual energy naturally. This part is very important and it is the basis of my method. Bear in mind you that there are natural ways to increase your energy without resorting to drugs and other devices that act only temporarily and have a lot of side effects.

The second part shows you how to control your ejaculation to last longer during the act of love.

These two parts go together party and you can not ignore one of them. The whole method will allow you to enjoy an exceptional sexuality!

In the space of a few weeks or a few months, depending on your commitment, you can transform your sex life. You'll be able to make love for 20, 30 minutes or hours without ejaculating. You also notice that your personality changes: you have more confidence in you; you know what you want from life. You will attract positive new circumstances and new positive people.

You need to think of your sexual energy as a seed that you plant. And this seed need to be given what it needs to grow. The same way you need to cultivate your sexual energy through a healthy lifestyle. It may take time but you won't have side effects.

First part :

Increase your sexual energy

Chapter 1:

Avoid Stress and pollution

Stress and pollution are two factors that can decrease your sexual energy .It is advisable not to make love when you are stressed.

There are several ways to fight against stress: meditation, yoga, exercise, and others. But one of the best ways is to sleep. Sleeping can recharge your sexual energy and allow you to cop well with the stress daily .Today many doctors recommend people to have 8-9 hours of sleep and to take naps .The Dalai Lama said "the best meditation is sleeping "staying late at night and not getting enough sleep could damage your sexual energy. So try to be stricter with your sleeping.

Also there is the pollution of the air and the electromagnetic waves that can really affect your body and reduce your testosterone level. Scientific studies show that better quality of air prolongs life; and everything that prolongs life increases sexual energy .If you live in the city, try to go parks every day for 20 minutes at least and during the holidays travel to the countryside or in the mountains to give energize your body and breathe fresh air. Fresh air is very important for your sexual energy; you can easily notice the good changes in your body when you spend some time in the fresh air: I am talking about days, or weeks.

Also never put your phone in your pockets near your testicles. In His book "the four hour body" author Tim Ferriss tells the anecdote of how he was shocked when he found out that his semen contained no sperm while he is a person who really takes care of his body. After research he realized that this was due to the phone that he put in his pockets. Two weeks after removing the phone from his pockets and his semen was back to normal. Put the phone in your briefcase or someplace else or otherwise hold it in your hand.

Rarely use the devices connected to the outlet .If you work with a computer, use the computer battery .Otherwise the connected computer (to the outlet) emits a very strong voltage (about 2 volts) which gives you feeling of being tired after using it .This voltage also decreases your sexual energy.

The impact of electromagnetic waves is not yet entirely clear to the scientific community .It is possible that this greatly reduces our sexual energy and we do not know it yet. By Precaution, use devices with the battery whenever you can.

Chapter 2:

Avoid harmful substances

By harmful substances, I think mainly cigarettes and alcohol, but it does exclude all other substances: cannabis, drugs...

Regarding smoking, I will not say much because health authorities are constantly reminding people: smoking kills you .But I will add that smoking reduces sexual force .So if you want to be a great lover reduce your cigarettes or stop it completely.

It is the same for alcohol. In his book "change your brain change your body," Dr. Amen request to avoid it completely because even the little glass of wine that you have while you eat could hurt your brain. A great lover avoids drinking alcohol either.

By the way, whenever you find an advice that will improve your brain, know that it will also improve your sexual energy.

Chapter 3:

A healthy diet

I can write another e-book about food, because of its importance for sexual energy.

First of all there's food to avoid the maximum and they are: sugar, white flour and salt. Brian Tracy the great guru of personal development called them: the three poisons .And unfortunately, they are everywhere. These three foods are very bad for the sexual energy.

You can replace sugar with: fruits, honey, maple syrup for example.

Select whole grains: brown rice, oat flakes, barley. Reduces your consumption of wheat and everything that is based on wheat like: pizzas... More and more doctors write books about the damage of wheat on the body and the brain .The wheat makes you fat and decreases sexual energy.

For salt: choose unrefined salt

Also avoid the chemicals in food: preservatives, colorings, aspartame, Chemicals starting with E and three digits (E333, E331 ...) or other any other code that they use in your country.

With whole grains, it is advised to eat a lot of vegetables especially raw vegetables: carrots, broccoli, cabbage (red white) spinach, radishes...

Add to it a little protein: white meat or fish or red meat.

Choose good oil: which contains lots of omega 3. Rape seed oil for cooking, and olive oil for seasoning or coconut oil. Avoid sunflower oil which contains omega 6, not good!

Oil consumption is important because it increases testosterone in men (as advocated by the author Tim Ferriss).

Daily consumption of coffee must be stopped replace it by tea.

If you suffer from problems such as premature ejaculation, frequent nocturnal ejaculations (one to two times per week) or impotence etc... I advise you to completely eliminate grains from your diet .and eat only vegetables and protein and lipids. Follow a paleo diet and your nocturnal ejaculation will stop.

Lipids or fats are very good for increasing sexual energy and cure premature ejaculation. The lipids stimulate sex hormones.

Among the best sources of fats: Olive oil, butter (preferably organic), coconut milk, coconut oil, avocado ...It is important to consume a certain amount of these lipids daily. Although we hear some say that fats are bad and they increase cholesterol, be aware that more and more experts recommend good sources of fat.

Of course, we must not confuse the good lipids (cited above) and bad fats such as: palm oil; hydrogenated oil ... that are often found in industrial food. The ideal is to follow a ketogenic diet (ketogenic diet) lipid based.

Moreover, daily consumption of vegetables helps increase energy .The raw vegetables contain more vitamins and minerals! Here is the basic food plan for a great lover. Try to follow it as much as you can.

There are also supplements that can boost your sexual energy. You can consume them regularly, or you can make cures of 1 month, 2 months, 3 months or more. You can consume them just before making love .These supplements are:

_ Ashwagandha: Plant from India known for giving the

"Strength of the horse", exists in powder. Ashwagandha is an aphrodisiac, boosts libido, cure impotence and fight against premature ejaculation, good for sperm.

_ Maca: it is a medicinal plant that is found mostly in powder form .It excellent aphrodisiac boosts virility; fight against sexual dysfunction, impotence, and give hard erections.

_The Ginseng: Root that stimulates virility, general tonic, increases confidence .cure impotence.

_ Tribulus terrestris: very powerful for its action on testosterone. Increases endurance, and physical strength (muscle gain) also good for fertility.

_ Royal jelly: gives strength, energy and vitality, combat impotence and frigidity.

_the pollen: Most often in the form of seeds, pollen is a natural tonic, increases vitality, fight against fatigue and activates spermatogenesis process in the testes.

There are other ways to increase sexual energy, such as: ginger; rhodiola; cinnamon; wolfberry; guarana; mandrake.

It is best to try them all (one by one), if possible, then see which one gives you more energy and more welfare or the one you like the most.

Chapter 4:

Physical exercise

Sport can increase your sexual energy as it can decrease it .All depends what sport you practice and how you do it. My advice is to first select a sport that you love; it can be the soccer game with friends, three yoga sessions per week or weight training sessions. The most important thing is to feel good at the end of the session. Second look for an activity that strengthens your body. Physical activity allows the secretion of dopamine (hormone of happiness, joy) in the brain .If you do not feel that you have more joy or more energy at the end of the session then it means that you need to do things differently and probably change activity.

In the context of this book program, it is recommended to do physical activity at least twice a week .The duration of a session can be from 7 to

30 min (intense session with 15 to 45 seconds of breaks). It is best to combine aerobic and anaerobic for instance cardio (running, for example) with weight training (Dead lift for example). Exercises that use the body weight are also good for increasing sexual energy push-ups, burpees, mountain climber....

This vigorous activity should be executed between 60% to 80% of your Maximum Heart Rate **(MHR)**

How to calculate your **MHR**:

a) - subtract your current age from 220. This number is your MHR.

b) - Multiply this number by 0.60. This is 60 percent of your MHR.

C) - take the number you came up with in step a). Multiply it by 0.80. This is 80 percent of your MHR.

These numbers of 60 percent and 80 percent represent the range of your Target Heart Rate (THR). (An important note: many high blood pressure medications work by lowering the heart rate, which would mean that your MHR and target rates may need to be lowered as well. If you are taking any blood pressure medications, contact your physician to find out how best to adjust these numbers).

When engaging in exercise, you will need to keep track of your heart rate to make sure you are staying within the 60 percent to 80 percent THR range. This is commonly done by lightly pressing the index finger of the right hand over the artery just under the skin on the skin on the inside of the left wrist. The rate is easily determined by counting the beats for 15 seconds, the multiplying that number by 4. This will be your heart rate. (Or count the beats for one minute).

If you don't like this way of counting your heart beats, there is an alternative rule of thumb: if you can hold a conversation, you aren't working hard enough. If you can sing, you are not working hard enough either. If you are out of breath, or have to stop and catch your breath, you're definitely working too hard. Stay in between!

Also it's important that you find an activity that you enjoy. There are a lot of activities out there, so find something that you enjoy.

Also where do you do your workout is very important .For example working out on the top of a mountain better than working out in a room, and that because the air quality is better on a mountain. So I recommend you to train outdoors in a park near a forest ... to get some fresh air. That is why you should focus on breathing for maximum energy intake.

If you like weight training I advise you three exercises that are best for increasing your energy, increasing your libido and regaining a perfect body:

_The Dead lift also allows you to work every muscle of the body including the back muscles. Great exercise for losing weight and strengthening the body.

_ The Bench press: it's a much known exercise. Allow you to work all the upper body (chest, shoulders, and arms).

_The Squat Very good exercise to work the legs, gluts and the abdominal belt.

Try to do these exercises at least twice a week to get results. You can find videos that explain you how to do them correctly.

Another exercise: stretching (stretching). Even if you cannot do a workout, stretch. It is good for strengthening the body and helps you lose weight.

Chapter 5:

Earthing!

Earthing, what does it mean?

Earthing is simply putting your feet (bare) on earth, or in direct contact with the earth, Connecting to ground. This concept was recently discovered ; Scientifically it has been proven that the earth has energy and when you touch the ground, the energy enters the body and can repair, heal, increase energy ... Rossi, in his book "sex life of the foot and shoe," said that they found nerves on the feet associated with the reproductive organs. The more you practice Earthing and the more your libido increases.

To practice Earthing, I advise you to go in your garden or the nearest park from you (when it is not very cold) and put your feet on the ground (without shoes nor socks). You can even feel the energy of the earth invade your whole body (it's a nice feeling).

Daily practice of earthing for 20min could result in a significant increase in sexual energy. This practice is really important if you want to enjoy an active sexuality for years.

There is only one book "earthing" you can consult for more information about earthing.

Chapter 6:

The management
of energy expenditure.

The energy of your body is like money the more you save and the more you are "Rich" in sexual energy. If you spend the day working hard (physical or intellectual work), in the evening you come home to the house you turn on the TV and watch it for two or three hours, then you eat a big meal in the evening, then you make love with your partner then you will have spent a lot of energy.

If you do this for 330 days in a year so do not be astonish if you begin to have erectile dysfunction or suffer from impotence or premature ejaculation problems ... .These are just a message from your body that means you have exhausted your energy.

It depends on the body of each one. Know your body and your limits and take care of it .Today we live in a world where everything is done to make us loose energy. We are working more and more. We eat more of the wrong food (if you are not careful) .There is too much entertainment, too much pollution. Our Body and mind have no time to rest, that's why we have more health problems. So we have to manage our efforts and our energy expenditure:

_Take regular breaks during the day .5 to 10 minutes every hour.

_Rest on weekends (and don't spend it partying or drinking).

_ Sleep at night .Between 8 and 9 hours of sleep. Go to sleep early.

_ Take a vacation. Choose a place where you can relax, enjoy nature and recharge yourself.

_ Meditate for 20 minutes a day to calm your brain.

_ Do not abuse your sexual energy. Avoid ejaculating daily until you have learned the technique of ejaculation control. Again think of your sexual energy as money. When you don't have enough money you can't spend too much of it; you wait until you have more money. The same goes for your sexual energy. Limit your ejaculations in the beginning, so you can have more later.

Second part :

How to control your ejaculation

There is a muscle called the PC muscle located between your testicles and your anus .This muscle when contracted it can control not only the flow of urine but also ejaculation. You should know that every time you ejaculate, this PC muscle expands and weakens causing energy loss at that part.

To feel this muscle, you only have to urinate and then try to stop your urine. Your urine is stopped with the PC muscle.

Once you have recognized this muscle and you can feel it, you can start doing the exercise (it's only one exercise with many variations). The exercise is simply contracting the muscle again and again. At first it may seem boring but then things will be much but the results are worth it: you will be able to make love as much as you can.

You'll go through several steps:

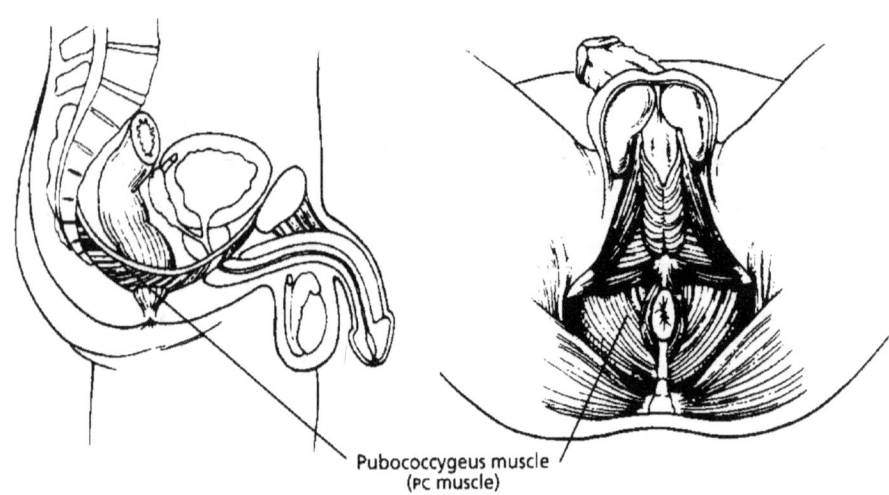

Pubococcygeus muscle
(PC muscle)

Step 1: Standing Contractions

In a standing position do the following contractions:

_Immediate Contraction/relaxation: the contraction lasts a second .The goal is to make the maximum of contraction in a given time

_ Contraction of 5 to 10 seconds: maintaining the contractions for 5 to 10 seconds.

_ Contraction of 1-2 minutes: maintaining the contraction for 1 to 2 minutes.

_ Long Contraction: long contractions can last 5 minutes, 10 minutes ... or more .you will feel the PC muscle burning a little and your leg might shake.

A session of 10 minutes a day can is what you need to get results and it will allow you to get to the next step.

You should not do all the variations in the same time or during a session. Start with one variation (for example: the immediate contractions) and do them for a week up to a month until you feel comfortable, then you can move to the next one.

Step 2: contraction in any position

After a while (about few weeks), you will be much more comfortable and your PC muscle will get stronger .you won't need to be standing to do the contractions, you'll be able to do them in any position: sitting, lying down ... you can watch TV while doing the exercises, that way you will not lose your time.

Try to do the same contractions of the first step but this time either sitting or lying down.

The transition from stage 2 to stage 3 can be done very quickly. You can walk while contracting your PC muscle. And even have a conversation holding the contraction.

Step 4: Contraction with an erect penis

The contraction with an erect penis is difficult compared to a flaccid penis .you must also train yourself with an erect penis .you will have to contract your PC muscle with more strength.

In this step, you should perhaps return to the standing position for better control of your contractions.

For steps 2-4 there is no time limit .you can do the exercises nonstop .you can do steps one by one or do them simultaneously. It all depends on your commitment to do the exercises.

Step 5: Contraction during the act of love.

This is the last step is the most difficult you will. Training to control your ejaculation as you want!

Conclusion

When you start to apply this method you will have to wait about three months (or more) to start having results. This is estimation; you can even have results after two months.

The first part is as important as the second, Always make sure that you are increasing your sexual energy.

Do not rush to make love before having well controlled your PC muscle, especially in Step 4 with the erect penis because during the act of love, you have so many distractions that you lose some control of your body.

Good luck!